Session Notes
NOTEBOOK

_____

_____

_____

D1318348

Client Details

NAME	CONTACT NO.	SESSION#	PAGE	NOTES

Client Details

NAME	CONTACT NO.	SESSION#	PAGE	NOTES

Date: _____ Start Time: _____ Session No: _____

Client Name: _____

Objective: _____

This Session Talking Key Points	Previous Session Talking Key Points

Notes:

_____
_____
_____
_____
_____
_____
_____
_____
_____
_____
_____
_____
_____
_____
_____
_____
_____
_____
_____
_____
_____
_____
_____

Extra Notes:

_____

_____

_____

_____

_____

_____

_____

_____

_____

_____

Client Actions	

Concerns	Recommendations

Comments:

_____

_____

_____

Next Session Topic & Discussion About	

Next Session Date: _____   End Time: _____

Date: _____   Start Time: _____   Session No: _____

Client Name: _____

Objective: _____

This Session Talking Key Points	Previous Session Talking Key Points

Notes:

_____
_____
_____
_____
_____
_____
_____
_____
_____
_____
_____
_____
_____
_____
_____
_____
_____
_____
_____
_____
_____
_____
_____
_____

Extra Notes:

_____
_____
_____
_____
_____
_____
_____
_____
_____
_____

Client Actions	

Concerns	Recommendations

Comments:

_____
_____
_____

Next Session Topic & Discussion About	

Next Session Date: _____   End Time: _____

Date: _____ Start Time: _____ Session No: _____

Client Name: _____

Objective: _____

This Session Talking Key Points	Previous Session Talking Key Points

Notes:

_____

_____

_____

_____

_____

_____

_____

_____

_____

_____

_____

_____

_____

_____

_____

_____

_____

_____

_____

_____

_____

_____

_____

Extra Notes:

_____
_____
_____
_____
_____
_____
_____
_____
_____
_____

Client Actions	

Concerns	Recommendations

Comments:

_____
_____
_____

Next Session Topic & Discussion About	

Next Session Date: _____   End Time: _____

Date: _____   Start Time: _____   Session No: _____

Client Name: _____

Objective: _____

This Session Talking Key Points	Previous Session Talking Key Points

Notes:

_____

_____

_____

_____

_____

_____

_____

_____

_____

_____

_____

_____

_____

_____

_____

_____

_____

_____

_____

_____

_____

_____

_____

Extra Notes:

_____
_____
_____
_____
_____
_____
_____
_____
_____

Client Actions	

Concerns	Recommendations

Comments:

_____
_____
_____

Next Session Topic & Discussion About	

Next Session Date: _____   End Time: _____

Date: _____ Start Time: _____ Session No: _____

Client Name: _____

Objective: _____

This Session Talking Key Points	Previous Session Talking Key Points

Notes:

_____
_____
_____
_____
_____
_____
_____
_____
_____
_____
_____
_____
_____
_____
_____
_____
_____
_____
_____
_____
_____
_____
_____

Extra Notes:

_____

_____

_____

_____

_____

_____

_____

_____

_____

_____

Client Actions	

Concerns	Recommendations

Comments:

_____

_____

_____

Next Session Topic & Discussion About	

Next Session Date: _____   End Time: _____

Date: _____   Start Time: _____   Session No: _____

Client Name: _____

Objective: _____

This Session Talking Key Points	Previous Session Talking Key Points

Notes:

_____
_____
_____
_____
_____
_____
_____
_____
_____
_____
_____
_____
_____
_____
_____
_____
_____
_____
_____
_____
_____
_____

Extra Notes:

_____
_____
_____
_____
_____
_____
_____
_____
_____
_____

Client Actions	

Concerns	Recommendations

Comments:

_____
_____
_____

Next Session Topic & Discussion About	

Next Session Date: _____   End Time: _____

Date: _____   Start Time: _____   Session No: _____

Client Name: _____

Objective: _____

This Session Talking Key Points	Previous Session Talking Key Points

Notes:

_____
_____
_____
_____
_____
_____
_____
_____
_____
_____
_____
_____
_____
_____
_____
_____
_____
_____
_____
_____
_____
_____
_____
_____

Extra Notes:

_____
_____
_____
_____
_____
_____
_____
_____
_____
_____

Client Actions	

Concerns	Recommendations

Comments:

_____
_____
_____

Next Session Topic & Discussion About	

Next Session Date: _____   End Time: _____

Date: _____   Start Time: _____   Session No: _____

Client Name: _____

Objective: _____

This Session Talking Key Points	Previous Session Talking Key Points

Notes:

_____
_____
_____
_____
_____
_____
_____
_____
_____
_____
_____
_____
_____
_____
_____
_____
_____
_____
_____
_____
_____
_____
_____

Extra Notes:

_____

_____

_____

_____

_____

_____

_____

_____

_____

_____

_____

Client Actions	

Concerns	Recommendations

Comments:

_____

_____

_____

Next Session Topic & Discussion About	

Next Session Date: _____   End Time: _____

Date: _____ Start Time: _____ Session No: _____

Client Name: _____

Objective: _____

This Session Talking Key Points	Previous Session Talking Key Points

Notes:

_____

_____

_____

_____

_____

_____

_____

_____

_____

_____

_____

_____

_____

_____

_____

_____

_____

_____

_____

_____

_____

_____

Extra Notes:

_____

_____

_____

_____

_____

_____

_____

_____

_____

_____

Client Actions	

Concerns	Recommendations

Comments:

_____

_____

_____

Next Session Topic & Discussion About	

Next Session Date: _____   End Time: _____

Date: _____   Start Time: _____   Session No: _____

Client Name: _____

Objective: _____

This Session Talking Key Points	Previous Session Talking Key Points

Notes:

_____
_____
_____
_____
_____
_____
_____
_____
_____
_____
_____
_____
_____
_____
_____
_____
_____
_____
_____
_____
_____
_____

Extra Notes:

_____

_____

_____

_____

_____

_____

_____

_____

_____

_____

Client Actions	

Concerns	Recommendations

Comments:

_____

_____

_____

Next Session Topic & Discussion About	

Next Session Date: _____   End Time: _____

Date: _____   Start Time: _____   Session No: _____

Client Name: _____

Objective: _____

This Session Talking Key Points	Previous Session Talking Key Points

Notes:

_____
_____
_____
_____
_____
_____
_____
_____
_____
_____
_____
_____
_____
_____
_____
_____
_____
_____
_____
_____
_____
_____
_____
_____

Extra Notes:

_____

_____

_____

_____

_____

_____

_____

_____

_____

Client Actions	

Concerns	Recommendations

Comments:

_____

_____

_____

Next Session Topic & Discussion About	

Next Session Date: _____   End Time: _____

Date: _____   Start Time: _____   Session No: _____

Client Name: _____

Objective: _____

This Session Talking Key Points	Previous Session Talking Key Points

Notes:

_____
_____
_____
_____
_____
_____
_____
_____
_____
_____
_____
_____
_____
_____
_____
_____
_____
_____
_____
_____
_____
_____

Extra Notes:

_____

_____

_____

_____

_____

_____

_____

_____

_____

Client Actions	

Concerns	Recommendations

Comments:

_____

_____

_____

Next Session Topic & Discussion About	

Next Session Date: _____   End Time: _____

Date: _____ Start Time: _____ Session No: _____

Client Name: _____

Objective: _____

This Session Talking Key Points	Previous Session Talking Key Points

Notes:

_____
_____
_____
_____
_____
_____
_____
_____
_____
_____
_____
_____
_____
_____
_____
_____
_____
_____
_____
_____
_____
_____
_____

Extra Notes:

_____
_____
_____
_____
_____
_____
_____
_____
_____
_____

Client Actions	

Concerns	Recommendations

Comments:

_____
_____
_____

Next Session Topic & Discussion About	

Next Session Date: _____   End Time: _____

Date: _____   Start Time: _____   Session No: _____

Client Name: _____

Objective: _____

This Session Talking Key Points	Previous Session Talking Key Points

Notes:

_____
_____
_____
_____
_____
_____
_____
_____
_____
_____
_____
_____
_____
_____
_____
_____
_____
_____
_____
_____
_____
_____

Extra Notes:

_____
_____
_____
_____
_____
_____
_____
_____
_____
_____

Client Actions	

Concerns	Recommendations

Comments:

_____
_____
_____

Next Session Topic & Discussion About	

Next Session Date: _____   End Time: _____

Date: _____   Start Time: _____   Session No: _____

Client Name: _____

Objective: _____

This Session Talking Key Points	Previous Session Talking Key Points

Notes:

_____
_____
_____
_____
_____
_____
_____
_____
_____
_____
_____
_____
_____
_____
_____
_____
_____
_____
_____
_____
_____
_____

Extra Notes:

_____
_____
_____
_____
_____
_____
_____
_____
_____
_____
_____

Client Actions	

Concerns	Recommendations

Comments:

_____
_____
_____

Next Session Topic & Discussion About	

Next Session Date: _____   End Time: _____

Date: _____   Start Time: _____   Session No: _____

Client Name: _____

Objective: _____

This Session Talking Key Points	Previous Session Talking Key Points

Notes:

_____

_____

_____

_____

_____

_____

_____

_____

_____

_____

_____

_____

_____

_____

_____

_____

_____

_____

_____

_____

_____

_____

_____

_____

_____

Extra Notes:

_____

_____

_____

_____

_____

_____

_____

_____

_____

_____

_____

Client Actions	

Concerns	Recommendations

Comments:

_____

_____

_____

Next Session Topic & Discussion About	
	-

Next Session Date: _____   End Time: _____

Date: _____ Start Time: _____ Session No: _____

Client Name: _____

Objective: _____

This Session Talking Key Points	Previous Session Talking Key Points

Notes:

_____
_____
_____
_____
_____
_____
_____
_____
_____
_____
_____
_____
_____
_____
_____
_____
_____
_____
_____
_____
_____
_____

Extra Notes:

_____
_____
_____
_____
_____
_____
_____
_____
_____
_____

Client Actions	

Concerns	Recommendations

Comments:

_____
_____
_____

Next Session Topic & Discussion About	

Next Session Date: _____   End Time: _____

Date: _____   Start Time: _____   Session No: _____

Client Name: _____

Objective: _____

This Session Talking Key Points	Previous Session Talking Key Points

Notes:

_____
_____
_____
_____
_____
_____
_____
_____
_____
_____
_____
_____
_____
_____
_____
_____
_____
_____
_____
_____
_____
_____
_____

Extra Notes:

_____
_____
_____
_____
_____
_____
_____
_____
_____
_____

Client Actions	

Concerns	Recommendations

Comments:

_____
_____
_____

Next Session Topic & Discussion About	

Next Session Date: _____   End Time: _____

Date: _____   Start Time: _____   Session No: _____

Client Name: _____

Objective: _____

This Session Talking Key Points	Previous Session Talking Key Points

Notes:

_____

_____

_____

_____

_____

_____

_____

_____

_____

_____

_____

_____

_____

_____

_____

_____

_____

_____

_____

_____

_____

_____

Extra Notes:

_____

_____

_____

_____

_____

_____

_____

_____

_____

_____

Client Actions	

Concerns	Recommendations

Comments:

_____

_____

_____

Next Session Topic & Discussion About	

Next Session Date: _____   End Time: _____

Date: _____   Start Time: _____   Session No: _____

Client Name: _____

Objective: _____

This Session Talking Key Points	Previous Session Talking Key Points

Notes:

_____
_____
_____
_____
_____
_____
_____
_____
_____
_____
_____
_____
_____
_____
_____
_____
_____
_____
_____
_____
_____

Extra Notes:

_____

_____

_____

_____

_____

_____

_____

_____

_____

_____

_____

_____

Client Actions	

Concerns	Recommendations

Comments:

_____

_____

_____

Next Session Topic & Discussion About	

Next Session Date: _____   End Time: _____

Date: _____ Start Time: _____ Session No: _____

Client Name: _____

Objective: _____

This Session Talking Key Points	Previous Session Talking Key Points

Notes:

_____

_____

_____

_____

_____

_____

_____

_____

_____

_____

_____

_____

_____

_____

_____

_____

_____

_____

_____

_____

_____

_____

_____

Extra Notes:

_____
_____
_____
_____
_____
_____
_____
_____
_____
_____
_____

Client Actions	

Concerns	Recommendations

Comments:

_____
_____
_____

Next Session Topic & Discussion About	

Next Session Date: _____   End Time: _____

Date: _____ Start Time: _____ Session No: _____

Client Name: _____

Objective: _____

This Session Talking Key Points	Previous Session Talking Key Points

Notes:

_____

_____

_____

_____

_____

_____

_____

_____

_____

_____

_____

_____

_____

_____

_____

_____

_____

_____

_____

_____

_____

_____

Extra Notes:

_____
_____
_____
_____
_____
_____
_____
_____
_____
_____

Client Actions	

Concerns	Recommendations

Comments:

_____
_____
_____

Next Session Topic & Discussion About	

Next Session Date: _____   End Time: _____

Date: _____ Start Time: _____ Session No: _____

Client Name: _____

Objective: _____

This Session Talking Key Points	Previous Session Talking Key Points

Notes:

_____
_____
_____
_____
_____
_____
_____
_____
_____
_____
_____
_____
_____
_____
_____
_____
_____
_____
_____
_____
_____
_____
_____
_____

Extra Notes:

_____
_____
_____
_____
_____
_____
_____
_____
_____

Client Actions	

Concerns	Recommendations

Comments:

_____
_____
_____

Next Session Topic & Discussion About	

Next Session Date: _____   End Time: _____

Date: _____ Start Time: _____ Session No: _____

Client Name: _____

Objective: _____

This Session Talking Key Points	Previous Session Talking Key Points

Notes:

_____
_____
_____
_____
_____
_____
_____
_____
_____
_____
_____
_____
_____
_____
_____
_____
_____
_____
_____
_____
_____
_____
_____

Extra Notes:

_____
_____
_____
_____
_____
_____
_____
_____
_____
_____

Client Actions	

Concerns	Recommendations

Comments:

_____
_____
_____

Next Session Topic & Discussion About	

Next Session Date: _____   End Time: _____

Date: _____   Start Time: _____   Session No: _____

Client Name: _____

Objective: _____

This Session Talking Key Points	Previous Session Talking Key Points

Notes:

_____
_____
_____
_____
_____
_____
_____
_____
_____
_____
_____
_____
_____
_____
_____
_____
_____
_____
_____
_____
_____
_____
_____

Extra Notes:

_____

_____

_____

_____

_____

_____

_____

_____

_____

_____

Client Actions	

Concerns	Recommendations

Comments:

_____

_____

_____

_____

Next Session Topic & Discussion About	

Next Session Date: _____   End Time: _____

Date: _____   Start Time: _____   Session No: _____

Client Name: _____

Objective: _____

This Session Talking Key Points	Previous Session Talking Key Points

Notes:

_____

_____

_____

_____

_____

_____

_____

_____

_____

_____

_____

_____

_____

_____

_____

_____

_____

_____

_____

_____

_____

_____

_____

Extra Notes:

_____

_____

_____

_____

_____

_____

_____

_____

_____

_____

Client Actions	

Concerns	Recommendations

Comments:

_____

_____

_____

Next Session Topic & Discussion About	

Next Session Date: _____   End Time: _____

Date: _____   Start Time: _____   Session No: _____

Client Name: _____

Objective: _____

This Session Talking Key Points	Previous Session Talking Key Points

Notes:

_____
_____
_____
_____
_____
_____
_____
_____
_____
_____
_____
_____
_____
_____
_____
_____
_____
_____
_____
_____
_____
_____
_____

Extra Notes:

_____

_____

_____

_____

_____

_____

_____

_____

_____

_____

Client Actions	

Concerns	Recommendations

Comments:

_____

_____

_____

Next Session Topic & Discussion About	

Next Session Date: _____   End Time: _____

Date: _____   Start Time: _____   Session No: _____

Client Name: _____

Objective: _____

This Session Talking Key Points	Previous Session Talking Key Points

Notes:

_____

_____

_____

_____

_____

_____

_____

_____

_____

_____

_____

_____

_____

_____

_____

_____

_____

_____

_____

_____

_____

_____

_____

Extra Notes:

_____

_____

_____

_____

_____

_____

_____

_____

_____

_____

Client Actions	

Concerns	Recommendations

Comments:

_____

_____

_____

Next Session Topic & Discussion About	

Next Session Date: _____   End Time: _____

Date: _____   Start Time: _____   Session No: _____

Client Name: _____

Objective: _____

This Session Talking Key Points	Previous Session Talking Key Points

Notes:

_____

_____

_____

_____

_____

_____

_____

_____

_____

_____

_____

_____

_____

_____

_____

_____

_____

_____

_____

_____

_____

_____

_____

_____

Extra Notes:

_____

_____

_____

_____

_____

_____

_____

_____

_____

Client Actions	

Concerns	Recommendations

Comments:

_____

_____

_____

Next Session Topic & Discussion About	

Next Session Date: _____   End Time: _____

Date: _____   Start Time: _____   Session No: _____

Client Name: _____

Objective: _____

This Session Talking Key Points	Previous Session Talking Key Points

Notes:

_____

_____

_____

_____

_____

_____

_____

_____

_____

_____

_____

_____

_____

_____

_____

_____

_____

_____

_____

_____

_____

_____

Extra Notes:

_____
_____
_____
_____
_____
_____
_____
_____
_____
_____
_____

Client Actions	

Concerns	Recommendations

Comments:

_____
_____
_____

Next Session Topic & Discussion About	

Next Session Date: _____   End Time: _____

Date: _____ Start Time: _____ Session No: _____

Client Name: _____

Objective: _____

This Session Talking Key Points	Previous Session Talking Key Points

Notes:

_____

_____

_____

_____

_____

_____

_____

_____

_____

_____

_____

_____

_____

_____

_____

_____

_____

_____

_____

_____

_____

_____

_____

_____

_____

Extra Notes:

_____

_____

_____

_____

_____

_____

_____

_____

_____

_____

Client Actions	

Concerns	Recommendations

Comments:

_____

_____

_____

Next Session Topic & Discussion About	

Next Session Date: _____   End Time: _____

Date: _____   Start Time: _____   Session No: _____

Client Name: _____

Objective: _____

This Session Talking Key Points	Previous Session Talking Key Points

Notes:

_____

_____

_____

_____

_____

_____

_____

_____

_____

_____

_____

_____

_____

_____

_____

_____

_____

_____

_____

_____

_____

_____

_____

Extra Notes:

_____

_____

_____

_____

_____

_____

_____

_____

Client Actions	

Concerns	Recommendations

Comments:

_____

_____

_____

Next Session Topic & Discussion About	

Next Session Date: _____   End Time: _____

Date: _____   Start Time: _____   Session No: _____

Client Name: _____

Objective: _____

This Session Talking Key Points	Previous Session Talking Key Points

Notes:

_____
_____
_____
_____
_____
_____
_____
_____
_____
_____
_____
_____
_____
_____
_____
_____
_____
_____
_____
_____
_____
_____
_____

Extra Notes:

_____
_____
_____
_____
_____
_____
_____
_____
_____
_____

Client Actions	

Concerns	Recommendations

Comments:

_____
_____
_____

Next Session Topic & Discussion About	

Next Session Date: _____   End Time: _____

Date: _____   Start Time: _____   Session No: _____

Client Name: _____

Objective: _____

This Session Talking Key Points	Previous Session Talking Key Points

Notes:

_____

_____

_____

_____

_____

_____

_____

_____

_____

_____

_____

_____

_____

_____

_____

_____

_____

_____

_____

_____

_____

_____

Extra Notes:

_____

_____

_____

_____

_____

_____

_____

_____

_____

Client Actions	

Concerns	Recommendations

Comments:

_____

_____

_____

Next Session Topic & Discussion About	

Next Session Date: _____   End Time: _____

Date: _____   Start Time: _____   Session No: _____

Client Name: _____

Objective: _____

This Session Talking Key Points	Previous Session Talking Key Points

Notes:

_____
_____
_____
_____
_____
_____
_____
_____
_____
_____
_____
_____
_____
_____
_____
_____
_____
_____
_____
_____
_____
_____
_____

Extra Notes:

_____

_____

_____

_____

_____

_____

_____

_____

_____

_____

Client Actions	

Concerns	Recommendations

Comments:

_____

_____

_____

Next Session Topic & Discussion About	

Next Session Date: _____   End Time: _____

Date: _____   Start Time: _____   Session No: _____

Client Name: _____

Objective: _____

This Session Talking Key Points	Previous Session Talking Key Points

Notes:

_____
_____
_____
_____
_____
_____
_____
_____
_____
_____
_____
_____
_____
_____
_____
_____
_____
_____
_____
_____
_____
_____
_____
_____

Extra Notes:

_____

_____

_____

_____

_____

_____

_____

_____

_____

_____

Client Actions	

Concerns	Recommendations

Comments:

_____

_____

_____

Next Session Topic & Discussion About	

Next Session Date: _____   End Time: _____

Date: _____ Start Time: _____ Session No: _____

Client Name: _____

Objective: _____

This Session Talking Key Points	Previous Session Talking Key Points

Notes:

_____
_____
_____
_____
_____
_____
_____
_____
_____
_____
_____
_____
_____
_____
_____
_____
_____
_____
_____
_____
_____
_____
_____
_____
_____
_____

Extra Notes:

_____

_____

_____

_____

_____

_____

_____

_____

_____

_____

Client Actions	

Concerns	Recommendations

Comments:

_____

_____

_____

Next Session Topic & Discussion About	

Next Session Date: _____   End Time: _____

Date: _____   Start Time: _____   Session No: _____

Client Name: _____

Objective: _____

This Session Talking Key Points	Previous Session Talking Key Points

Notes:

_____
_____
_____
_____
_____
_____
_____
_____
_____
_____
_____
_____
_____
_____
_____
_____
_____
_____
_____
_____
_____
_____
_____

Extra Notes:

_____

_____

_____

_____

_____

_____

_____

_____

_____

_____

Client Actions	

Concerns	Recommendations

Comments:

_____

_____

_____

Next Session Topic & Discussion About	

Next Session Date: _____   End Time: _____

Date: _____ Start Time: _____ Session No: _____

Client Name: _____

Objective: _____

This Session Talking Key Points	Previous Session Talking Key Points

Notes:

_____
_____
_____
_____
_____
_____
_____
_____
_____
_____
_____
_____
_____
_____
_____
_____
_____
_____
_____
_____
_____
_____
_____
_____

Extra Notes:

_____
_____
_____
_____
_____
_____
_____
_____
_____
_____

Client Actions	

Concerns	Recommendations

Comments:

_____
_____
_____

Next Session Topic & Discussion About	

Next Session Date: _____   End Time: _____

Date: _____   Start Time: _____   Session No: _____

Client Name: _____

Objective: _____

This Session Talking Key Points	Previous Session Talking Key Points

Notes:

_____
_____
_____
_____
_____
_____
_____
_____
_____
_____
_____
_____
_____
_____
_____
_____
_____
_____
_____
_____
_____
_____

Extra Notes:

_____

_____

_____

_____

_____

_____

_____

_____

_____

_____

Client Actions	

Concerns	Recommendations

Comments:

_____

_____

_____

Next Session Topic & Discussion About	

Next Session Date: _____   End Time: _____

Date: _____ Start Time: _____ Session No: _____

Client Name: _____

Objective: _____

This Session Talking Key Points	Previous Session Talking Key Points

Notes:

_____

_____

_____

_____

_____

_____

_____

_____

_____

_____

_____

_____

_____

_____

_____

_____

_____

_____

_____

_____

_____

_____

_____

Extra Notes:

_____
_____
_____
_____
_____
_____
_____
_____
_____
_____

Client Actions	

Concerns	Recommendations

Comments:

_____
_____
_____

Next Session Topic & Discussion About	

Next Session Date: _____   End Time: _____

Date: _____   Start Time: _____   Session No: _____

Client Name: _____

Objective: _____

This Session Talking Key Points	Previous Session Talking Key Points

Notes:

_____

_____

_____

_____

_____

_____

_____

_____

_____

_____

_____

_____

_____

_____

_____

_____

_____

_____

_____

_____

_____

_____

Extra Notes:

_____

_____

_____

_____

_____

_____

_____

_____

_____

_____

Client Actions	

Concerns	Recommendations

Comments:

_____

_____

_____

Next Session Topic & Discussion About	

Next Session Date: _____   End Time: _____

Date: _____ Start Time: _____ Session No: _____

Client Name: _____

Objective: _____

This Session Talking Key Points	Previous Session Talking Key Points

Notes:

_____

_____

_____

_____

_____

_____

_____

_____

_____

_____

_____

_____

_____

_____

_____

_____

_____

_____

_____

_____

_____

_____

_____

_____

Extra Notes:

_____

_____

_____

_____

_____

_____

_____

_____

_____

_____

Client Actions	

Concerns	Recommendations

Comments:

_____

_____

_____

Next Session Topic & Discussion About	

Next Session Date: _____   End Time: _____

Date: _____ Start Time: _____ Session No: _____

Client Name: _____

Objective: _____

This Session Talking Key Points	Previous Session Talking Key Points

Notes:

_____
_____
_____
_____
_____
_____
_____
_____
_____
_____
_____
_____
_____
_____
_____
_____
_____
_____
_____
_____
_____
_____
_____

Extra Notes:

_____

_____

_____

_____

_____

_____

_____

_____

_____

_____

_____

Client Actions	

Concerns	Recommendations

Comments:

_____

_____

_____

Next Session Topic & Discussion About	

Next Session Date: _____   End Time: _____

Date: _____ Start Time: _____ Session No: _____

Client Name: _____

Objective: _____

This Session Talking Key Points	Previous Session Talking Key Points

Notes:

_____
_____
_____
_____
_____
_____
_____
_____
_____
_____
_____
_____
_____
_____
_____
_____
_____
_____
_____
_____
_____
_____
_____
_____

Extra Notes:

_____

_____

_____

_____

_____

_____

_____

_____

_____

_____

_____

Client Actions	

Concerns	Recommendations

Comments:

_____

_____

_____

Next Session Topic & Discussion About	

Next Session Date: _____   End Time: _____

Date: _____   Start Time: _____   Session No: _____

Client Name: _____

Objective: _____

This Session Talking Key Points	Previous Session Talking Key Points

Notes:

_____

_____

_____

_____

_____

_____

_____

_____

_____

_____

_____

_____

_____

_____

_____

_____

_____

_____

_____

_____

_____

_____

Extra Notes:

_____

_____

_____

_____

_____

_____

_____

_____

_____

_____

Client Actions	

Concerns	Recommendations

Comments:

_____

_____

_____

Next Session Topic & Discussion About	

Next Session Date: _____   End Time: _____

Date: _____ Start Time: _____ Session No: _____

Client Name: _____

Objective: _____

This Session Talking Key Points	Previous Session Talking Key Points

Notes:

_____

_____

_____

_____

_____

_____

_____

_____

_____

_____

_____

_____

_____

_____

_____

_____

_____

_____

_____

_____

_____

_____

_____

_____

_____

Extra Notes:

_____

_____

_____

_____

_____

_____

_____

_____

Client Actions	

Concerns	Recommendations

Comments:

_____

_____

_____

Next Session Topic & Discussion About	

Next Session Date: _____   End Time: _____

Date: _____   Start Time: _____   Session No: _____

Client Name: _____

Objective: _____

This Session Talking Key Points	Previous Session Talking Key Points

Notes:

_____

_____

_____

_____

_____

_____

_____

_____

_____

_____

_____

_____

_____

_____

_____

_____

_____

_____

_____

_____

_____

_____

_____

Extra Notes:

_____
_____
_____
_____
_____
_____
_____
_____
_____
_____

Client Actions	

Concerns	Recommendations

Comments:

_____
_____
_____

Next Session Topic & Discussion About	

Next Session Date: _____   End Time: _____

Date: _____ Start Time: _____ Session No: _____

Client Name: _____

Objective: _____

This Session Talking Key Points	Previous Session Talking Key Points

Notes:

_____
_____
_____
_____
_____
_____
_____
_____
_____
_____
_____
_____
_____
_____
_____
_____
_____
_____
_____
_____
_____
_____
_____

Extra Notes:

_____
_____
_____
_____
_____
_____
_____
_____
_____
_____

Client Actions	

Concerns	Recommendations

Comments:

_____
_____
_____

Next Session Topic & Discussion About	

Next Session Date: _____   End Time: _____

Date: _____ Start Time: _____ Session No: _____

Client Name: _____

Objective: _____

This Session Talking Key Points	Previous Session Talking Key Points

Notes:

_____
_____
_____
_____
_____
_____
_____
_____
_____
_____
_____
_____
_____
_____
_____
_____
_____
_____
_____
_____
_____
_____
_____
_____

Extra Notes:

_____

_____

_____

_____

_____

_____

_____

_____

_____

_____

Client Actions	

Concerns	Recommendations

Comments:

_____

_____

_____

Next Session Topic & Discussion About	

Next Session Date: _____   End Time: _____

Date: _____   Start Time: _____   Session No: _____

Client Name: _____

Objective: _____

This Session Talking Key Points	Previous Session Talking Key Points

Notes:

_____

_____

_____

_____

_____

_____

_____

_____

_____

_____

_____

_____

_____

_____

_____

_____

_____

_____

_____

_____

_____

_____

_____

_____

Extra Notes:

_____

_____

_____

_____

_____

_____

_____

_____

_____

_____

Client Actions	

Concerns	Recommendations

Comments:

_____

_____

_____

Next Session Topic & Discussion About	

Next Session Date: _____   End Time: _____

Date: _____ Start Time: _____ Session No: _____

Client Name: _____

Objective: _____

This Session Talking Key Points	Previous Session Talking Key Points

Notes:

_____
_____
_____
_____
_____
_____
_____
_____
_____
_____
_____
_____
_____
_____
_____
_____
_____
_____
_____
_____
_____
_____
_____
_____

Extra Notes:

_____
_____
_____
_____
_____
_____
_____
_____
_____
_____

Client Actions	

Concerns	Recommendations

Comments:

_____
_____
_____

Next Session Topic & Discussion About	

Next Session Date: _____   End Time: _____

Date: _____ Start Time: _____ Session No: _____

Client Name: _____

Objective: _____

This Session Talking Key Points	Previous Session Talking Key Points

Notes:

_____
_____
_____
_____
_____
_____
_____
_____
_____
_____
_____
_____
_____
_____
_____
_____
_____
_____
_____
_____
_____

Extra Notes:

_____

_____

_____

_____

_____

_____

_____

_____

_____

_____

Client Actions	

Concerns	Recommendations

Comments:

_____

_____

_____

Next Session Topic & Discussion About	

Next Session Date: _____   End Time: _____